# HEALTH SERVICES MANAGEMENT

## Competition and Co-operation

### A way to improve health sector performance

# HEALTH SERVICES MANAGEMENT

---

# Competition and Co-operation

## A way to improve health sector performance

---

## A REPORT
### Prepared by Grant Thornton Management Consultants

THE NUFFIELD
PROVINCIAL HOSPITALS TRUST

Published by the
Nuffield Provincial Hospitals Trust
3 Prince Albert Road, London NW1 7SP

ISBN 0 900574 62 3
© Nuffield Provincial Hospitals Trust, 1986

Designed by Bernard Crossland
PRINTED IN GREAT BRITAIN BY
BURGESS & SON (ABINGDON) LTD
ABINGDON OXFORDSHIRE

# CONTENTS

Editorial Note                                                    vii

Preface                                                             3

**The Study Background,** 3. The Study and it's Aims, 3. The Study Report
and Handbook, 3. **Report Summary,** 4. Main Conclusions, 4. The Nature
of Co-operation, 5. The Alternative Ways of Developing Co-operation, 6.
The Changes Required to the NHS, 7. The Wider Importance of the
Changes to the NHS, 8. The Private Sector Size and Capability, 9. Private
Sector Developments, 10. Conclusion, 11.


## PART I Public Sector Developments

1 NHS Internal Market Transactions                                15

Introduction, 15. Shortcomings in the Present NHS Arrangements for
Inter Unit Transfers, 15. The Elements of an Internal Market Transaction
System, 17. Competitive Tendering and an Internal Market System, 18.

2 Financial Structure and Reporting                               20

Introduction, 20. Management Difficulties Caused by Present Financial
Arrangements, 21. Moving to a Devolved Basis of Management, 23.

3 NHS Capital Asset Accounting                                     25

Introduction, 25. The Need for NHS Capital Asset Accounting, 25. The
Necessary Elements of a Capital Accounting System, 26.

4 NHS Revenue Earning Activities                                   28

Introduction, 28. Short-term Selling of Services, 28. Long-term Selling of
Services, 29. Long-term Selling of NHS Private Beds and Treatment, 29.
Changes needed to the management of NHS private beds, 30. Long-term
Selling of NHS Skills and Services other than Pay Beds, 32. The
development and investigation of opportunities, 33. Management and
profitability of services sold on a long-term basis, 34. The role of the
consultant in long-term sale of services, 35.

## PART II **Private Sector Developments**

5 Private Sector Size and Coverage                    39

Introduction, 39. Summary of Conclusions Relating to the Size of the
Private Sector, 39. The Overall Provision of Acute Beds, 41.
Conclusion, 43. The Regional Provision of Facilities, 43. Conclusions, 45.
Hospital Ownership, Size and Service Provision, 45. Conclusion, 47.

6 Specific Service Provision by the Private Sector    49

Introduction, 49. Summary of Conclusions, 49. Data Collection, 50.
Pathology Service, 51. Conclusion, 52. Pharmacy Services, 53.
Conclusions, 55. X-Ray Diagnosis and Treatment Services, 55.
Conclusions, 56.

7 Private Sector Developments                         58

Introduction, 58. The Encouragement of Selected Growth Areas, 58.
Regulation of the Private Sector, 60. The present arrangements for
regulation, 60. Aspects of self-regulation in the private health sector, 61.

## PART III **Programme and Conclusion**

8 A Suggested Programme                               67

Introduction, 67. Immediate Developments, 67. Longer Term
Developments, 69.

9 Conclusion                                          70

# EDITORIAL NOTE

In 1984 the Trust, following a commission to Thornton Baker Associates, now Grant Thornton, Management Consultants, published the results of a study of competitive tendering in the provision of domestic, catering, and laundry services, in the form of a Practical Guide and Handbook.

Subsequently, the Trust commissioned Grant Thornton to carry out a further study into the potential for co-operation between the public and private health sectors, in the clinical field of acute treatment and medical services.

In the event, the Trustees have decided to publish the report of this study in two parts, since in effect it conveniently divides between what might generally be called issues of policy, and observations which are suitable for a practical guide and handbook which deals with those practical questions concerned with the development of co-operation between public and private hospitals.

This monograph, the first part of the report, falls naturally into the Occasional Paper series of the Trust being concerned with the more fundamental issues concerned with policy. It deals with the nature of co-operation, the alternative ways of developing it and certain changes which are required to maximise the effect of the resources available in each sector for the improvement of health services in general. It thus provides basic material for the discussion of long-term policy, an essential stage in policy-making to distinguish the myths from the facts and it is hoped help dispel many of the confusions which bedevil the public and private mix of health services.

*Acknowledgements*
The Trustees wish to thank Mr Peter Cuthbert-Smith and Mr Jeremy Noble of Grant Thornton, who carried out the survey and

produced the report; also the Managers in the NHS and the private sector who so willingly assisted the Grant Thornton team.

G.McL

3 Prince Albert Road
London NW1
*May 1986*

# HEALTH SERVICES MANAGEMENT

## Competition and Co-operation

### A way to improve health sector performance

# PREFACE

## The Study and its Aims

1. The Nuffield Provincial Hospitals Trust has been involved for a number of years in research into the potential for co-operation between the U.K. public and private health care sectors. In 1982 the Trust published a major study—*The Public/Private Mix for Health,* and then in 1983 commissioned Thornton Baker Associates, (now called Grant Thornton, Management Consultants) to prepare a Practical Guide and Handbook concerning competitive tendering in the provision of hospital domestic, catering and laundry services.

2. Since that time, the debate about the public/private sector for health has continued and in 1985 the NPHT asked Grant Thornton to make a further study. The purpose of this second study was to consider co-operation between the public and private health sectors in relation to patient treatment and medical services.

3. The study takes as its base the present position in which two separate health sectors exist side by side, both with valuable resources and skills. The study explores the question of how the two sectors might operate a policy of co-operation as a means of obtaining best use of their resources in the overall provision of the country's health care. The study has concentrated on the acute sector in England but many of its conclusions will also be relevant in other aspects of health care, and other parts of the U.K.

## The Study Report and Handbook

4. The study began by reviewing the co-operative ventures which have already taken place between the two sectors, and discussing the general

3

needs of such ventures with senior management. From these discussions the team prepared a series of guidelines, setting out the lessons to be learnt from the existing practice, and providing general suggestions for the way in which co-operative arrangements should be set up. These detailed results of the study are being published by the Trust separately from this report as a Practical Guide and Handbook called *Developing co-operation between Public and Private hospitals.*

5. It was clear to the team that there were a number of important and fundamental matters relating to the NHS and to the private sector where major change would be needed before a policy of co-operation could be operated at anything other than at a relatively low level. It was decided that these more fundamental issues should be discussed in a separate publication, and that is the purpose of this report.

---

## REPORT SUMMARY

---

## Main Conclusions

1. The study's main conclusions about the nature of co-operation between the public and private health sectors in the U.K. are:

(1) Co-operation between the two health sectors means the buying and selling of health care services and patient treatment between hospitals on a basis which takes financial and commercial matters fully into account.

(2) The adoption of a policy of co-operation would tend to create a market for buying and selling services between the two sectors and also between NHS hospitals; such a market would have many of the competitive features associated with commercial markets and would provide pressure for cost reduction, better use of resources and innovation generally.

(3) The full development of co-operation and its associated market would require important changes in the financial and accounting arrange-ments for health authorities to put them in a position where they have

increased freedom and motivation to enter into competitive buying and selling arrangements with the private sector.

(4) The changes required in health authority financial and accounting arrangements would not alter the basis nature of the NHS as a provider of free health care; the changes are, however, of fundamental importance in improving management performance and require careful consideration even if a policy of co-operation is not adopted.

(5) The private sector, although not large in comparison with the public sector, is judged to be of sufficient size to enable a policy of co-operation to be initiated.

(6) The development of co-operation will require a strong and growing private sector; the sector may require encouragement to develop in certain geographical areas and specialisms and, more importantly, the sector needs to consider its methods for self-regulation in order to ensure that it maintains sound standards.

2. These conclusions are described more fully in the remainder of this Preface.

## The Nature of Co-operation

3. In practical terms, co-operation between the public and private health sectors means the buying and selling of surplus capacity and specialist services between public health authorities and private sector organisations. Managements in many industries use this kind of buying and selling of capacity and services in order to achieve their objectives and to obtain the optimum utilisation of their resources.

4. The use of the word 'co-operation' to describe purchase and sale agreements of this kind is perhaps misleading. It may imply arrangements made for the common good with little concern for the financial realities of the situation. In the past, there may have been charities and religious organisations which worked without particular regard for financial matters. Now, however, the main organisations making up the private sector, although many of them may be registered as charities or mutual groups, must necessarily have close regard to the financial and commercial aspects of their activities if they are to continue in their work.

5. This means that co-operation between the two sectors will have to be on a basis which takes financial and commercial matters fully into account. It means, in particular, that in setting up co-operative arrangements the NHS and private sector organisations will both try to negotiate the lowest possible prices for the services they wish to buy, and that both will attempt to earn maximum revenue for the skills and services they have available for sale to each other. The development of co-operation between the two sectors thus concerns the development of trading arrangements in what will have many of the characteristics of a commercial market.

## The Alternative Ways of Developing Co-operation

6. There is a decision to be made regarding the way in which co-operation between the two sectors is to be dealt with. One option would be to allow the present approach to be continued, in which co-operation arrangements are set up on a relatively infrequent and informal basis. This approach has undoubtedly been a useful one and the study found a number of interesting co-operative ventures which have already taken place. It is, however, an approach which essentially retains the present sharp division between the two sectors and which in the longer term would be limited in what it could achieve.

7. The alternative option would be to encourage the concept of co-operation to develop into a more dynamic form of working relationship between the two sectors. In many ways, this would be a natural development because as already explained the financial pressures which now exist in both sectors mean that the buying and selling of services would tend to create something approaching a market between hospitals. The existence of a market of that kind would provide an environment in which competition and innovation could develop.

8. Initially such a market might operate at two levels. At one level, which can be called the 'external' market, private operators would sell both services and patient treatment to NHS hospitals and NHS hospitals would sell services to private hospitals. At the second level, in what has been called an 'internal market', NHS hospitals would enter into buying and selling arrangements with each other for both patient treatment and

services. Clearly, over a relatively short period of time the external and internal markets would tend to converge with both being influenced by the same competitive pressures.

9. The development of a combined market of that kind would have an important effect on the management of both sectors. Private sector management would have to take account of the opportunities which a larger market would offer together with increasing competition in that market from the NHS. NHS management would have to develop in a way which allowed it to operate within a more competitive environment and to make use of the purchase and sale of services as a means of improving overall performance.

10. This alternative approach towards co-operation would not change the essential nature of the NHS, although a number of very important changes would have to be made to enable it to operate in a way which would allow a more open market to be developed. The private sector, although expanding, is relatively small at present and would also need to develop in a number of ways if it was to play an effective role in such a market and take advantage of the opportunities it offered.

## The Changes Required to the NHS

11. The changes in NHS management which it would be necessary to make if this approach were adopted are described in Part I of this report. First, there are the changes which would be needed to develop an internal market within the NHS by devising a mechanism by which health authorities can enter into buying and selling arrangements with each other, in competition with the services available from the private sector. The elements of the charging systems which would be needed to do this are described in Chapter 1.

12. The second area in which changes in the NHS would be needed relate to the financial and accounting arrangements. If the aim is to encourage health authorities to look for innovative arrangements with the private sector and with other NHS units, then it is necessary to provide them with increased freedom and incentive to do so, and it is necessary to be able to monitor the results they achieve. Meeting these needs will involve

increasing the financial autonomy of health authorities together with their responsibility for achieving objectives. This will require the introduction of a revised form of legal accounts for each authority, based on the use of statements of assets, liabilities and income and expenditure. The proposed changes to financial and reporting arrangements are outlined in Chapter 2.

13. The NHS operates from an extensive base of capital assets. With the continuing application of technology to medicine the amount of financial resources to be applied to capital assets is likely to become even more significant than at present. However, health authorities have no means of accounting for assets or for measuring their use in financial terms. As part of putting the financial arrangements onto a basis on which authorities can more effectively be held responsible for their financial results, it will be necessary to develop comprehensive asset accounting systems. These are discussed in Chapter 3.

14. Finally, in order to enable health authorities to operate effectively in competition with the private sector, it will be necessary to clarify the financial and management arrangements for those NHS activities used to earn revenue. It will be necessary for these to operate on a sound commercial basis if maximum revenue is to be earned by the NHS, and fair competition between the NHS and the private sector is to be maintained. The proposals for dealing with NHS revenue earning activities are given in Chapter 4.

## The Wider Importance of the Changes to the NHS

15. The proposed changes to the NHS are those needed to enable a policy of co-operation between the two sectors to be fully developed. However, the proposed changes have a far wider importance than that of developing inter-sector co-operation.

16. The NHS is providing a sophisticated service to meet individual patient's needs, and is working in an environment of advanced and rapidly developing technology. The effective management of health authority resources must rank as one of the most complex and difficult tasks faced by management in any organisation. The present financial

structure and reporting arrangements for health authorities are those based on the general accounting principles used by government departments. These principles are effective in controlling departments which carry out a relatively straightforward and unchanging activity, but are generally less well suited to the management of complex organisations such as health authorities.

17. For this reason, it is difficult to see how health authorities can improve their performance generally without changes to the financial and reporting systems being made of the kind described in this report. For example, it is difficult to see how performance can be improved without there being a means for recording assets in health authority accounts and without management being made financially responsible for the efficient use of those assets. Similarly, it is difficult to see that without an effective means for making transfers of cost between authorities to meet cross-boundary flows of patients and services, management can control and be held responsible for use of resources. Without a means of accounting for revenue earning activities on a commercial basis, it is difficult to see that management can be satisfied that their revenue earning activities are financially viable.

18. It is therefore emphasised that there is a fundamental need for changes of this kind in the financial and management arrangements of health authorities which is of greater importance than that of being able to operate a policy of inter-sector co-operation. That wider need should be borne in mind, and such changes given serious consideration even if a policy of increased co-operation between the sectors is not adopted.

## The Private Sector Size and Capability

19. Turning now to the private sector, the study team's first aim was to assess whether the private sector as it currently exists in the U.K. was of a size where it could provide the basis for the development of co-operation on a reasonable scale.

20. The private sector is diverse, with many different types and size of operation varying from the charitable and mutual organisations to the 'for profit' companies. The statistical work of the study shows that in

overall terms the private sector provides some 6 per cent of all acute beds in England and thus remains relatively small when compared to the total resources of the NHS. However, when particular types of operation are considered, the private sector provides a far more significant contribution and for certain conditions may provide up to 20 per cent of all elective surgery. Geographically, private sector hospitals tend to be concentrated in the Thames regions, but there is some degree of private sector facility in all English health regions. There has been a general growth in the sector in recent years, with a trend towards larger units offering a range of services and operating facilities.

21. In general terms, therefore, the team considered that the private sector's size is sufficient to provide a small but adequate basis on which to initiate a policy of co-operation between the two sectors.

## Private Sector Developments

22. A policy of co-operation between the two sectors will become increasingly effective the larger the private sector becomes and the wider the range of services it offers. The study was not concerned with identifying the general conditions for future growth of the private sector, but two aspects were considered in relation to the development of co-operation.

23. The first of these aspects is the encouragement of those growth areas in the private sector which would be important in the context of co-operation. It may well be possible through the use of planning agreements between health authorities and private sector units to encourage growth in particular ways, for example growth in particular geographical areas, or growth in particular specialisations and in new ways of providing health care. Further suggestions for areas where growth might be stimulated are given in Chapter 7.

24. The second aspect of the private sector considered during the study was its regulation. There is a need for any industry or service to maintain the confidence of the consumer. Where health is concerned, the consumer must have total confidence in the provider. At the present time, the private health sector would generally be judged to enjoy an extremely

high level of confidence and nothing in the present study has indicated otherwise. Even so, if the market is to grow, with possibly new operators joining it, it may well be advisable for the private sector to take steps to ensure that this confidence level is maintained and that it has the mechanism available to do so. If, for example, general confidence in the private sector was for any reason to fall, the general growth of the market for the private sector would be seriously inhibited and, in particular, it would become very difficult for the NHS to enter into co-operation arrangements.

25. At present, the regulation of private health sector hospitals is provided by local health authorities, carrying out the responsibility placed on them by legislation. This regulation covers the registration and inspection of premises, and deals with the physical and technical aspects of hospital operation. The private sector should now consider the development of a form of self-regulation to deal with the qualitative and business aspects of their activities as a means of making sure that the sector retains its present high reputation and consumer confidence. Self-regulation is discussed in Chapter 7.

## Conclusion

26. The concept of co-operation between the two sectors is thus far wider than it appears at first sight. It could be used as a means for creating a more open market for services and treatment with the stimulation of competition and freedom for innovation which such markets provide. No change in the essential nature of the NHS as a provider of free health care would be required. Important changes to financial and management reporting for health authorities would however be needed as part of a general strengthening of management's control. Private sector management should give careful consideration to the regulation of their sector to provide a sound basis for their future growth.

# PART I
# Public Sector Developments

# CHAPTER 1

# NHS Internal Market
# Transactions

## Introduction

1. The selling of surplus capacity and the buying in of services to meet demand are important in enabling management to maximise the use of its resources. It is management practices of this kind which will provide the main driving force behind the development of co-operation between the public and private health sectors.

2. However, from the point of view of a unit manager in the NHS, it would be possible to maximise the use of resources by buying and selling services within the rest of the NHS equally as well as by buying and selling services within the private sector. Hence the importance of the concept of developing a system for dealing with internal market transactions within the NHS to operate in conjunction with the development of arrangements for buying and selling with the private sector.

## Shortcomings in the Present NHS Arrangements for Inter Unit Transfers

3. At present there are no generally adopted arrangements for making charges between districts or regions for the transfer of services or patients. Where such arrangements exist, they tend to be based on an annual charge calculated at the end of the year on the basis of cost sharing. Alternatively, adjustments may be made in subsequent funding allocations to take account of cross-boundary flows. But, even if they are made, any adjustments of that kind will tend to be retrospective, and will clearly not enable the provider of the service to be recompensed until one or two years after the event.

4. In practical terms therefore there is no comprehensive system for inter authority charging in the NHS for the cross-boundary flows of patients and services. Specifically, this means that:

(1) There is no mechanism by which a management can sell surplus capacity to another district and receive revenue for the sale within the financial year.

(2) There is no mechanism by which management using the resources of another district will be charged with the costs of those resources in the financial year.

5. The consequences of this lack of a system for making inter authority transfers are important in the effective management of the NHS. It means that there can be no really effective way for monitoring management's overall use of resources, and there may well be an incentive not to manage resources in the most efficient way. For example, if a surplus capacity arises in a particular authority, there is no incentive for management to make that capacity available to other NHS authorities—they would receive no extra revenue for doing so, and might well incur additional costs; there may thus be an incentive not to make spare capacity available. For similar reasons, management seeking to obtain additional capacity may find it difficult to find a seller of that capacity within the NHS.

6. A more general example of the consequences of the lack of an inter authority transfer system relates to the provision of specialist services and skills. For example, a particular hospital may develop a specialist skill, or require an advanced piece of specialist equipment. Such skills and equipment may well attract transfer patients from many other authorities, for which the hospital providing the service will incur additional costs, but will receive no additional revenue. The hospital providing the advanced skills thus comes under severe cost pressure, while the authorities from which the patients are sent suffer no loss of revenue and benefit by their lack of initiative in developing their own specialist services.

7. The ultimate position would arise when the hospital providing the specialist service had no more funds and had to cease operations until the

next year's funds allocation was received. High quality resources would thus become unutilised for a period, which might well have been used by other parts of the NHS, if inter authority charging had been possible.

8. The lack of a comprehensive system for internal market transfers in the NHS is thus an important restriction on management which:

(1) Provides no means for encouraging management to use all surplus NHS capacity.

(2) Restricts management's ability to purchase services from within the NHS.

(3) Provides a disincentive to become a centre of excellence or to provide a specialist service.

(4) Does not penalise managements which make ineffective use of resources.

(5) Provides no means for transfer of funds to those authorities which are providing an effective service which is in demand.

## The Elements of an Internal Market Transaction System

9. The aim of developing an internal market system within the NHS would be to enable services to be 'bought' and 'sold' between districts at 'market' prices. It might be necessary to develop certain rules regarding internal pricing and transfer mechanism but, the aim should be that from the point of view of a unit manager, the internal NHS market and the external private sector market should appear to be similar, with both offering similar opportunities for effective buying and selling. In this way an element of competition can be introduced into the internal system without making any change to the essential nature of the NHS as a provider of free health care.

10. There need to be two principal elements in an internal market transaction system for the NHS:

(1) The first element is a system for charging for patients who are transferred across boundaries. To do this, the present system of

recording hospital activity needs to be developed so that it can form the basis for calculating the charges to be made to the unit or district from which the patients came. Although charges would be based on negotiation, they would need to be supported by clinical budgeting and patient costing systems. An internal market system for patient charging is therefore probably for longer term development because its general adoption would require the introduction of a number of major new systems. However, there would appear to be no reason why special 'one off' arrangements should not be negotiated now for patient transfer, possibly using standard cost data.

(2) The second element of an internal market system is the procedures for inter authority charging for services bought and sold between hospitals. There would seem to be no reason why the costs of these services could not be calculated now sufficiently accurately to allow for inter authority charging for services to be introduced in the immediate future.

## Competitive Tendering and an Internal Market System

11. The concept of competitive tendering has an important part to play within the operation of an internal market system for the NHS. Competitive tendering involves seeking tenders for a service from outside contractors and also from the provider of the existing in-house service. The in-house and external tenders are compared and the tender with the lowest cost is accepted.

12. The concept of competitive tendering would form an essential part of an internal market system, with tenders being obtained from other NHS units or districts, as well as from the existing in-house providers and from the external private sector. The concept could be operated now in relation to services.

13. More importantly, however, it seems likely that competitive tendering could be operated now in relation to patient waiting lists. Where a district has an unacceptable waiting list for a particular treatment it would be possible for a number of cases to be made the subject of a competitive

tendering process in which NHS and private sector hospitals would be allowed to bid.

14. It is suggested that funds might be made available to districts to be used specifically for reduction of certain waiting lists. It could be stipulated that those funds could be spent only by means of competitive tendering involving both private hospitals and NHS hospitals. In addition to achieving a reduction in waiting lists, an initiative of this kind would make an effective way to introduce the concepts of internal market transfers into the NHS.

# CHAPTER 2

# NHS Financial Structure
# and Reporting

## Introduction

1. The present financial structure and reporting arrangements for the NHS are based on the normal financial and accounting bases used by government departments and government related bodies which operate by means of funds provided from a central government source. The general principle on which these financial arrangements operate is that of public funds being voted for spend on certain closely defined activities. In general, such funds must be spent on the matters for which they were voted, and spent within the financial year. Only a strictly limited amount of movement of funds between activities is permitted, and only a limited amount of unspent funds can be carried forward from one year to the next.

2. Public financing and accounting arrangements of this kind have served the public sector well, and are effective in controlling the spending of departments carrying out a relatively straightforward activity which changes little from year to year. Where, however, the activities become more complex and where flexibility is required, financial arrangements of this kind tend to restrict the organisation concerned from being operated effectively.

3. The management of the NHS is a complex matter which comes within this category. The effective management of NHS resources to achieve optimum utilisation is as complex and difficult a task as the management of any large business or public sector organisation. But, the present NHS financial and reporting arrangements tend to restrict the ability of management in their role; by concentrating on a rigid control of specified expenditure, the present financial arrangements substantially reduce

management's ability to be flexible and to manage their resources in the optimum way.

4. Increasingly in the public sector, the approach has been to try new ways of overcoming the rigidity of public sector financial and accounting arrangements in order to enable management to manage flexibly and effectively while remaining within public sector control. The purpose of this chapter is to examine how this might be achieved within the NHS as a means of helping management to operate effectively and to be in a better position for co-operation and competition with the private sector.

## Management Difficulties Caused by Present Financial Arrangements

5. The present financial arrangements for the NHS are based on the annual RAWP allocations of funds for revenue and capital spend, the application of strict expenditure control and the application of cash limits.

6. The RAWP allocations of funds to districts are made by central government and distributed by regional authorities. The RAWP is an allocation formula based on population considerations. Once awarded, funds are not passed to districts in the form of lump sum payments to be managed by district management. Instead, funds have to be requisitioned by districts as required when expenditure is incurred.

7. During the year, district management controls expenditure precisely to the agreed levels of spend. Considerable management effort has to be made to ensure that cash limits are not exceeded, and that all funds are used during the year and are not 'lost' through being unable to carry unspent funds forward to a following year.

8. Authorities will receive expenditure statements during the year and the formal legal financial returns are prepared at the year end. These consist of detailed analyses of expenditure under certain predetermined headings, but provide no statement of assets. Considerable amounts of statistical cost data are collected with the aim of being able to compare one authority with another and to provide performance indicators to provide a means for measuring service performance.

9. Financial systems of this kind provide a highly effective means for controlling spend, but they provide little assistance to management in their task of managing resources effectively to achieve the overall aims of their organisation. From a management point of view, the principal shortcomings of the present financial and reporting arrangements in the NHS are:

(1) Management's freedom to use the funds made available to them is restricted; they can spend funds only in accordance with a predetermined budget which tends to restrict their ability to be flexible and to initiate new activities.

(2) The system is such that it tends to force management's time horizon to be the end of the current financial year; the need to control expenditure so very closely within the financial year takes a considerable proportion of management's time, and inhibits the ability to take cost decisions which affect future years.

(3) The present legal accounts of authorities do not include any statement of assets; management is not therefore put in a position of having to be responsible for asset management which, considering the high technology and consequent high value of many NHS assets, is an essential aspect of management.

(4) The absence of responsibility for asset and funds management means that an authority and its management has no incentive to manage its resources on a continuing basis with the aim of building up its asset base, retaining surplus funds and generally increasing the 'wealth' of the district or region.

(5) There is no statement of income and expenditure which incorporates charges for assets, there is thus no effective basis on which to enter into buying and selling arrangements with the private sector, or to control the use of resources in internal market transfer arrangements with other districts.

(6) There is a misconception that the production of statistical cost and performance data will assist management to manage resources effectively; effective management can happen only when the responsibilities of individual managers are identified and cost data is reported according to those responsibilities and is fully integrated with the overall financial and reporting arrangements.

## Moving to a Devolved Basis
## of Management

10. It should be possible to overcome the restrictions on management of the present financial and reporting arrangements and move towards a position in which local management would be given a far higher level of responsibility for managing the affairs of their authority and in which they would be given considerably increased flexibility in their powers to manage. Such an approach would be consistent with the general philosophy behind the recent appointment of general managers in the NHS.

11. The aim would be to put authorities on a more independent basis, while retaining overall government control over policy and while retaining the essential nature of the NHS. To do this, authorities would have to be put into a position in which they become far more responsible than at present for their own financial affairs and for managing those affairs in the best way to achieve the policy objectives of patient care which have been set for them. Increasing authorities' responsibilities for their own financial affairs would be a means for building on management's sense of proprietorship which can be an important motivation element in management.

12. An important aspect of increasing authorities' responsibility for their own financial affairs is that it would necessarily involve management in the competitive buying and selling of services between NHS units, districts and regions, as well as with the private sector. Once management is given financial responsibility it can no longer permit cross-boundary flows of patients and services without payment. The giving of financial responsibility would result in competitive buying and selling as a means of improving financial performance.

13. The principal elements which would have to form the basis of a devolved form of financial and reporting structure for the NHS are:

(1) Overall policy would be set by central government and regional management as at present, with quantified aims and objectives for each authority to meet being set in terms of the levels of patient care

which are required. Authorities' performance would be measured against these targets.

(2) Authorities would have to move towards a financial basis on which they would be provided with a fixed annual grant from government, and would be able to raise external finances within certain controlled limits. Authorities would be allowed to retain unspent grants, and surpluses on sales of assets. Deficits would have to be made good by authorities out of future annual grants.

(3) Authorities would be given the power to make investments; this would include short-term investment of funds, investment in subsidiary companies, and investment in joint ventures with the private sector.

(4) The formal legal accounts of an authority would consist of a balance sheet and income and expenditure statements; the balance sheet should record all assets, normal depreciation policies should apply and authorities should be allowed to hold reserves.

(5) Districts' accounts should be consolidated at regional level for submission to central government.

(6) Activities entered into by districts for profit (such as pay beds) would be put into separate trusts or subsidiary companies and be given normal commercial targets for financial return. Profits from those activities would be used by the authorities who would also have to deal with any losses incurred.

(7) All pricing of services sold by authorities would be on a full commercial basis, with the same arrangements being applied to sales and purchases within the NHS and to the private sector.

14. Due to the unique nature of the services provided by the NHS, such arrangements would probably be as far as it is possible to develop the NHS financial and management structure in the direction of autonomy and competition, while retaining the overall nature of the NHS and overall government control.

# CHAPTER 3

# NHS Capital Asset Accounting

## Introduction

1. At present the NHS operates no system of capital asset accounting. Funds are allocated for capital spend and are used on agreed capital projects. The expenditure is charged in the year in which it is incurred but there is no means for recording in the accounting systems the value of the capital asset.

2. The question of capital assets has been explored recently by the CIPFA capital and asset accounting working party and reported on in their report *Managing Capital Assets in the National Health Service* (May 1985). The purpose of this chapter is to consider the relevance of capital accounting in the context of co-operation with the private sector and the general developments in the NHS discussed in this part of the report.

## The Need for NHS Capital Asset Accounting

3. The NHS makes use of an extensive range of existing assets and each year commits major new capital expenditure. The development of medical technology means that health authorities will increasingly use equipment and buildings which are technically specialised and high cost. The effective management of this very complex and high cost asset base is a major and difficult task.

4. At present, NHS management have little financial information to help them in making sure that fully effective use is being made of these assets. There is no means of showing asset values in the accounts, with the result that managers have no knowledge in financial terms of the capital resource which they are managing, and so cannot be held responsible for its effective management. The users of NHS assets, namely the heads of

departments and doctors, have no charge made to their department for the use they make of capital equipment and buildings and so cannot be held responsible for the effective usage of those assets.

5. The lack of capital asset accounting means that a major piece of capital equipment could be seriously under-utilised with there being no financial penalty placed on the department concerned. In this case, there would be no financial incentive on management to improve utilisation by internal users, to sell the surplus capacity to external users, to replace the equipment with an alternative, or to dispose of the equipment and put the funds to a better use.

6. There is thus an important need for a capital asset accounting system in the internal management of NHS resources. The need also exists in considering private sector co-operation and the buying and selling of services within the NHS. The lack of capital asset accounting in this context means that it is difficult to arrive at the full comparative cost of the internal services when deciding whether to purchase services from a private operator or from another unit. Equally, it is difficult to ensure that the sales price of any NHS services being offered to the private sector includes capital costs.

7. More important, however, is the consideration that in many cases the purchasing of services from the private sector, or from another NHS unit, involves what can be called a 'trade-off' between capital and revenue expenditure. For example, a proposed arrangement with another operator may mean a high initial capital investment with low future revenue expenditure as opposed to continuing with the high revenue expenditure of the existing in-house arrangement. The look of capital asset accounting in the NHS means that management has no incentive to develop such 'trade-offs'.

## The Necessary Elements of a Capital Accounting System

8. The operation of a capital accounting system is thus an essential part of developing the health authorities' management of their assets and more importantly would be an essential part of putting authorities into a

position in which they are responsible for managing their own financial affairs.

9. In this context, the main elements which would have to be incorporated in a capital accounting system would be:

(1) Each authority would have to record all capital assets and their cost.

(2) Each authority would prepare an annual balance sheet in which are included capital assets.

(3) A depreciation charge for all assets would be included as part of the income and expenditure statement to be prepared for each authority.

(4) The depreciation charge should be included in departmental costs.

(5) Authorities should be given greater flexibility to sell assets, (including sales to other NHS units), profit or loss on sale being the responsibility of the authority and remaining in the authority's accounts.

10. Details of the recording of capital assets, and the way in which this should be done in the NHS have been provided in some detail in the CIPFA report referred to earlier, and will not be repeated here.

# CHAPTER 4

# NHS Revenue Earning Activities

## Introduction

1. This chapter deals with those activities which health authorities undertake in order to earn additional revenue to assist in supporting their other services. The chapter deals with revenue earning from pay beds and from the sale of NHS skills and resources. Clearly, if health authorities are to be able to operate effectively in co-operation and competition with the private sector it is essential that they have the means to manage and account for their revenue earning activities on a sound commercial basis.

2. The use of NHS facilities for sale to the private sector has been the subject of political and social debate over many years. This report is not concerned with that debate, but views the sale of such services as a management task. From a purely management point of view, if the NHS has resources and skills which can be sold then it is a valid management practice to sell these services as a means of generating further revenue to be used for the main objectives which have been set. Clearly, however, management should not allow the selling of such services to direct their efforts from the fundamental purposes of the NHS.

## Short-term Selling of Services

3. Short-term selling situations arise when managers see they have short-term surplus capacity and they try to sell that capacity to another user at a price which shows a surplus over the marginal cost of providing the service. By its nature, short-term surplus capacity may only last for a few days or weeks, and may arise at short notice. It therefore normally requires a rapid decision-making process, and is best carried out at operational management level.

4. Within the NHS, there would appear to be no reason why operational

level management in charge of departments should not be encouraged to sell short-term surplus capacity in this way. This will require the operation of the clinical budgeting systems which are currently being developed within the NHS. No other developments in the financial or management systems will be needed.

## Long-term Selling of Services

5. Long-term selling occurs when an organisation takes a policy decision to enter a given market on a permanent basis, and acquires assets and resources specifically with the intention of using them to provide a service at a full commercial profit with an adequate return on capital.

6. Within the NHS, long-term sales positions can arise in two main instances:

(1) The provision of pay beds to private patients.

(2) The sale of specialist skills and services.

7. The development of a sound and commercially based approach to those two types of revenue earning activity will be important in putting the NHS into a position from which it can compete with the private sector through the commercial purchase and sale of services. Both topics are discussed in the remainder of this chapter.

## Long-term Selling of NHS Private Beds and Treatment

8. When the NHS provides beds for private patients it enters fully into the private sector market. It is then in direct competition with private hospitals, and is not working in co-operation with them.

9. In practice the fact that NHS pay bed activities are an integral and important part of the private sector market does not always seem to be recognised in the way this part of the service is operated and sold, and in particular, full advantage does not seem to be taken of the revenue potential from this source.

10. The charges to be made for NHS private beds are fixed nationally for the UK as a per diem charge covering all services including drugs and implants. Charges are not varied according to location, services rendered or the particular circumstances relating to individual hospitals.

11. Separate accounts for the pay bed activity are not normally prepared, and the assets and resources used are not separately identified. For the larger private wings a separate administrator may be appointed, but in general the post of commercial manager with responsibility for the commercial and financial viability of the private bed activity does not exist.

### Changes needed to the management of NHS private beds

12. Viewed from the management point of view there are a number of important shortcomings in the present arrangements for the provision of private beds by the NHS. These will have to be overcome if this activity is to generate maximum net income for the NHS, provide effective competition and form an innovatory force in the health sector in general.

13. The shortcomings in the present arrangements centre around the point that although operating fully in the private market, the NHS pay bed activities are not set up on a commercially oriented basis. In particular:

(1) There are no financial targets for the return on capital to be earned from the activity.

(2) The relevant assets and other resources used in the activity are not identified, and no separate accounts are prepared to enable success to be judged.

(3) Management has not been given the responsibility for managing the activity on a commercial basis.

(4) The considerable technical strengths of the medical resources supporting the service do not appear to be exploited through the pricing arrangements; the centralised fixing of prices does not allow effective pricing decisions to be taken at the operational level.

14. There are a number of fundamental changes which are needed to put the NHS pay bed activity onto a sound commercial basis. Of those changes, the most important one would be for districts, and units to separate pay bed activity from their normal NHS operations. The separation might be achieved by putting the activity into a separate division, trust or company, with its own accounting and financial records. A useful further development might be for other private operators to be invited to take shares in the new subsidiary company which would enable effective joint venture and management contracts to be developed between the two sectors.

15. Once the concept of separating out the private bed activities from the main NHS activities has been accepted, it is possible to see how the activity could be operated in an effective commercial way for the ultimate benefit of the NHS:

(1) The DHA and RHA would have to develop a policy for their pay bed activity and decide on the amount of investment and financial return they needed.

(2) Management would be appointed to the new pay bed subsidiary with the responsibility for the commercial management of the activity and would be set financial targets for return on investment.

(3) The assets required for the activity on a full-time basis would be transferred at a valuation into the new pay bed subsidiary.

(4) The new subsidiary would have to meet its own operating costs, and would be charged on a full commercial basis for all services provided by the NHS.

(5) Management would fix charges to patients at the price they considered was the market price, bearing in mind their responsibility to earn a financial return.

(6) The new subsidiaries would be self financing; profit surplus to requirements could be paid to the DHA.

(7) Losses could only be financed by the DHA on normal commercial loan arrangements. DHA's would have to be prevented from meeting trading losses as part of their normal expenditure.

(8) The relationship between the management of the pay bed subsidiary and the consultants would be the same as the one which exists in the private sector.

16. The setting up of NHS pay bed activity on an 'arms length basis' in this way would allow the activity to be managed effectively, on a full commercial profit basis. All charges between the NHS and the pay bed subsidiary would be at full commercial rates, and all profits would go to the NHS. It would allow the NHS to play a more effective part in the private sector, providing, and being subject to, powerful competition. It would provide an effective base for the NHS to take the lead in innovation in the private sector.

## Long-term Selling of NHS Skills and Services other than Pay Beds

17. As explained earlier in this chapter, the selling of skills and services on a long-term basis is different in concept from the selling of short-term spare capacity which is only a means of improving short-term resource utilisation. Long-term selling of services means entering a market on a full-time commercial basis, and means committing assets and other resources specifically for that purpose. The entering into long-term selling arrangements requires a formal decision by senior management after proper investigation to ensure that the arrangement will be a valid commercial enterprise and will generate surplus revenue over the life of the project.

18. A number of districts have entered into long-term markets in areas other than pay beds and examples are the provision of pathology services and pharmacy to private sector hospitals. Joint ventures, where there is agreement to share costly equipment may also come within this context. All long-term selling arrangements of this kind are important within the context of co-operation between the two sectors, and in the provision of additional sources of revenue for the NHS.

19. There are however two important aspects of long-term selling arrangements which need to be considered:

(1) the range, development and investigation of opportunities;

(2) the management and profitability of the services being sold.

## The development and investigation of opportunities

20. The range and depth of technical skills and knowledge available in the NHS, including those of the consultants, is second to none. In addition to serving NHS patients, it may well be that many of these specialist technical skills and 'know-how' are marketable in the UK and overseas context. However, few of these skills appear to be being used to develop additional revenue for the NHS, and few case studies of actual selling arrangements have been located during this study.

21. It is therefore suggested that authorities should consider appointing a commercial manager, who should be responsible to the general manager for developing the business activities of the authority on a basis which is commercially viable and shows an adequate financial return on investment for the authority. The role of the commercial manager should be to:

(1) Assess the particular specialist skills and services available within the authority.

(2) Review the external markets available to the authority (which should include other health authorities).

(3) Make fully costed proposals to the authority for entering suitable markets on a fully commercial basis.

(4) Develop the authority's activities in those markets on a financially viable basis.

22. The role of the commercial manager, and a suggested development programme to be followed is given in the practical guide which the Nuffield Provincial Hospitals Trust is publishing separately from this report. The way in which the sale of services should be financed and managed is discussed below.

**Management and profitability of services sold on a long-term basis**

23. It has already been explained that when services are sold on a long-term basis, it means that specific assets and other resources are allocated permanently to that activity. Such resources have to be financed on a permanent basis and interest on the capital required has to be paid. For these reasons, when a decision is taken to enter into the market or service arrangement on a long-term basis, the financial criteria have to be based on the full costs of the activity, including capital funding. The sale prices agreed for the activity have to be such that over a period they will recover all these costs and yield an adequate return on the funds employed.

24. In the NHS at present, the systems and financial structure are such that it is extremely difficult to cost on a full commercial basis an activity which is being sold on a long-term basis. In particular it is difficult to cost the staff and services provided to the activity, and probably impossible to arrive at the capital value of the assets being used. The concern is that any expansion of the sale of services in the way described in this chapter might be implemented on a basis which did not recover all costs and earn a true surplus for NHS use. Clearly, unless adequate surpluses can be demonstrated, management should not be entering into long-term sales arrangements.

25. It is suggested that consideration should be given by authorities to putting any activity which is engaging in long-term selling to a private market into a separate operating division, or separate subsidiary company, on similar lines to that proposed earlier for pay beds. The creation of separate operating divisions or companies to deal with long-term commercial activities would mean that such activities were segregated, from other operations. They would have to be self accounting and would have to identify and cost all resources and assets used. A required return on assets could be specified and charges for services would have to be calculated on a commercial basis to earn the necessary return. The manager of the new division or company would have the responsibility for earning that return.

**The role of the consultant in long-term sale of services**

26. This study has not been concerned with the arrangements relating to the employment and remuneration of consultants in the NHS. At a number of points, however, these arrangements have a connection with the management matters which are the concern of the study. One of those matters concerns the role of the consultant in any long-term selling arrangements of the kind discussed above.

27. In many cases, an NHS service which is marketable on a long-term basis may well be lead by a consultant who is in charge of the service and who provides technical supervision, with non-consultant staff managing the service on a day-to-day basis. If the NHS is to be in a sound position when negotiating long-term sales arrangements with outside organisations it has to be such that the service being provided includes the technical and other supervision of the consultants in charge of the activity. Any arrangement in which a 'customer' had to negotiate once with the NHS for the service and a second time with the consultant for the supervision of the service is unlikely to be viable from a business or management point of view. It is unlikely that such an arrangement could be made to be profitable from the point of view of generating surplus revenue for the NHS on a full commercial basis. It is therefore concluded that all arrangements by the NHS to enter markets permanently with a view to making long-term sales contracts, must include all the consultant's technical and specialist skills required as part of the service being provided.

# PART II

# Private Sector Developments

# CHAPTER 5

# Private Sector Size and Coverage

## Introduction

1. An important part of the study was the investigation of the size of the private sector to assess whether it was large enough and sufficiently broadly based to provide an adequate response should the NHS adopt a policy of increased co-operation. In this chapter, the overall size of the private sector is considered in relation to beds and to geographical spread. In the following chapter, the range of private sector services is examined, and then in the final chapter of Part II the need for changes in the private sector is considered.

## Summary of Conclusions Relating to the Size of the Private Sector

2. In reviewing the private sector the team has collected and examined data from a range of published sources. The main conclusions which can be drawn from the data are summarised below. In each case the conclusion and relevant data are discussed in more detail in the paragraphs indicated:

(1) **The overall provision of acute beds** (Paragraphs 3 to 8)

The findings suggest that although in total the private sector is small in relation to total NHS resources, it appears to be of sufficient size to provide the basis for a policy of developing co-operative arrangements for the performance of elective surgery.

(2) **Regional provision of facilities** (Paragraphs 9 to 11)

The findings suggest that although the major concentration of private hospitals continues to be in the Thames regions, all English regions now have some degree of local private sector facility for elective surgery with which to conclude short- and long-term co-operative arrangements. The geographical spread of private facilities should enable most DHAs to involve private hospitals in competitive tendering procedures.

(3) **Hospital ownership, size, and service provision** (Paragraphs 12 to 17)

The findings suggest that the expansion in acute hospital facilities during the last six years has produced larger units in terms of average number of beds. The expansion in size of private hospital units increases the potential for co-operative ventures in health care.

TABLE 1. *NHS and Private Sector Acute Beds*

| Health Region | (a) NHS Beds Acute Specialities | (b) Private Acute Beds (Excluding NHS Pay Beds) |
|---|---|---|
| Northern | 10230 | 144 |
| Yorkshire | 11514 | 537 |
| Trent | 11509 | 500 |
| East Anglia | 5197 | 272 |
| N.W.T | 9677 | 1238 |
| N.E.T | 13450 | 1692 |
| S.E.T | 11117 | 823 |
| S.W.T | 7665 | 977 |
| Wessex | 7285 | 604 |
| Oxford | 5702 | 470 |
| S. West | 8993 | 430 |
| W. M | 14493 | 529 |
| Mersey | 7545 | 282 |
| N. West | 13216 | 616 |
| Total | 137593 | 9114 |
| Percentage of all Acute Beds | 94% | 6% |

*Notes*
(a) Average daily available beds 1983. *Source:* Health Personal Social Services Statistics (DHSS), Tables 1;2 and 4;9.
(b) Source AIH and Grant Thornton 1985.

## The Overall Provision of Acute Beds

3. In performing the data collection and analysis for the study the team have used a number of sources of data including published and unpublished material from trade associations and government, and where necessary the team has carried out specific exercises to collect data. The collection and review of the data requires careful definition of terms; the definition of acute hospitals and beds used by the team throughout the study has been:

'Hospitals providing in-patient care, equipped with operating facilities, but excluding hospitals and beds wholly or mainly dedicated to abortion, long-term geriatric care or elective cosmetic surgery.'

4. Table 1 shows the number of private sector acute beds (excluding NHS pay beds) compared to available NHS beds in acute specialities by health

TABLE 2. *Acute Bed Provision Per Population*

| Region | Private Acute Beds per 1000 of Population (Excluding NHS Pay Beds) | NHS Acute Staffed Beds Per 1000 of Population | Private Sector as % of Total |
|---|---|---|---|
| Northern | 0·05 | 3·3 | 1·5 |
| Yorkshire | 0·15 | 3·2 | 4·5 |
| Trent | 0·11 | 2·5 | 4·2 |
| East Anglia | 0·16 | 2·7 | 5·6 |
| N.W.T | 0·37 | 2·8 | 12·0 |
| N.E.T | 0·43 | 3·6 | 10·6 |
| S.E.T | 0·23 | 3·1 | 6·9 |
| S.W.T | 0·33 | 2·6 | 11·3 |
| Wessex | 0·21 | 2·6 | 7·5 |
| Oxford | 0·20 | 2·4 | 7·7 |
| S. West | 0·13 | 2·9 | 4·3 |
| W. M | 0·11 | 2·8 | 3·8 |
| Mersey | 0·12 | 3·1 | 3·7 |
| N. West | 0·15 | 3·3 | 4·3 |

*Sources:* Grant Thornton 1985 and DHSS: Health and Personal Social Services Statistics 1983.

region. This data shows that the private acute sector provided approximately 6 per cent of total acute beds in 1983 in England.

5. A further measure of the private sector size when compared to the NHS is to relate bed availability to resident population. This gives a more meaningful assessment of the potential contribution to acute health care in specific regions than absolute numbers of beds. Table 2 shows the number of beds per 1000 of population in each health region. Examination of the data shows that, depending on region, the private sector (excluding NHS pay beds) contributed between 1 per cent to 12 per cent of total acute beds in England in 1983.

6. Several commentators have suggested that the size of the private sector relative to the NHS as measured by data given in Tables 1 and 2 is not a fully adequate measure of its contribution to health care. For this reason Nicholl and colleagues (*Lancet,* July 1984) analysed all elective inpatient

TABLE 3. *Selected Operations by Sector of Treatment*

|  | Percentage of Operations Performed | |
|---|---|---|
|  | *Per cent Private Sector Plus NHS Pay Beds* | *Per cent Private Sector Only* |
| Tonsillectomy and Adenoidectomy | 14·5 | 9·3 |
| Hernia Repair | 14·0 | 10·0 |
| Haemorrhoidectomy | 23·7 | 20·2 |
| Cholecystectomy | 11·0 | 7·6 |
| Hysterectomy | 20·9 | 17·6 |
| Hip Replacement | 26·2 | 16·4 |
| Excision Knee Structure | 22·8 | 16·9 |
| Varicose Veins | 23·0 | 18·9 |
| All other operations | 12·3 | 9·8 |
| All elective surgery (Excluding abortion) | 13·2 | 9·8 |

*Source:* Nicholl, *et al.* (*Lancet,* July 14 1984) and Grant Thornton, 1985.
*Note:* Data refers to residents of England and Wales.

operations performed in 148 private hospitals in 1981 on residents in England and Wales and compared these with the NHS pay bed and non-pay bed admissions data from the Hospital Inpatient Enquiry (HIPE) records. Table 3 shows the results of this analysis. It lists eight types of operation which were common on NHS waiting lists and which represented nearly 25 per cent of private hospital activity.

7. The analysis in Table 3 shows that the proportion of the eight sampled operations performed in the independent hospital and NHS pay bed sectors ranges from 11 to 26 per cent of all operations in these eight categories performed in the NHS and private sector combined. If NHS pay beds are excluded, the proportion of these operations performed wholly in the private sector ranges from 7·6 to 20 per cent. Table 3 also indicates that overall nearly 10 per cent of all elective surgery in England and Wales is performed wholly in the private sector.

**Conclusion**

8. In 1979 the Royal Commission on the National Health Service concluded that apart from abortions the scale of private treatment was too small to make a significant impact on the NHS. The data presented above suggests that the position has changed since then and that the private sector now makes a more significant contribution to all elective surgery performed in England. In particular operations where consider-able waiting lists exist in the NHS this contribution appears to be of even greater significance. Since the study by Nicholl and colleagues was performed significant growth in the private sector has taken place and as a result the contribution to elective surgery may well also have shown a parallel growth trend, although this has not been investigated by the study team.

# The Regional Provision of Facilities

9. Historically the provision of private acute facilities has been concen-trated in the South-East regions. The initial development of private hospitals in close proximity to the London teaching hospitals was a factor in this situation. During the period 1979 to 1985 development continued

in the South-East but a significant expansion in facilities also occurred elsewhere in England. This expansion reflected the local demand for private facilities resulting from wider medical insurance cover of the resident population. Table 4 shows that the private hospital sector has added 63 units since 1979. This growth of approximately 58 per cent over the 1979 number has been largely in the provision of hospital facilities

TABLE 4. *Regional Growth in Private Hospital Facilities*

| | No. of Hospitals 1985 | New Private Hospital Units Since 1979 | New Hospital Beds as a % of Regions Total Private Beds 1985 |
|---|---|---|---|
| **London Regions** | | | |
| N.W.T | 14 | 6 | 37 |
| N.E.T | 24 | 6 | 15·6 |
| S.E.T | 16 | 6 | 39·4 |
| S.W.T | 15 | 5 | 25·5 |
| S/Total | 69 | 23 | |
| % of Total | 40% | 36% | |
| **Other Regions** | | | |
| Northern | 3 | 2 | 45·8 |
| Yorkshire | 14 | 5 | 30 |
| Trent | 13 | 4 | 31·4 |
| East Anglia | 8 | 2 | 36·7 |
| Wessex | 14 | 8 | 62·2 |
| Oxford | 12 | 5 | 47·8 |
| S. West | 10 | 3 | 23 |
| W. Midlands | 14 | 4 | 40·2 |
| Mersey | 5 | 2 | 34·4 |
| N. West | 10 | 5 | 37·2 |
| S/Total | 103 | 40 | |
| % of Total | 60% | 64% | |
| Total No. of Hospitals | 172 | 63 | |
| Total % Growth over 1979 | | 58% | |

*Source:* AIH and Grant Thornton.

outside the London regions. Table 4 shows that 40 new hospitals or 64 per cent of the total added between 1979 to 1985 have been in the ten non-London regions. In all the 14 regions of England there are now private acute facilities.

10. Further analysis performed by the team into the location of private hospitals in district health authorities showed that 119 out of the 191 DHAs (62 per cent) now have a private acute hospital within their boundaries, 35 out of these 119 DHAs (29 per cent) have more than one private hospital present within the district. Of those DHAs with no private facility in their district, only four authorities do not now have a private hospital in an adjoining district in the same region or a neighbouring region.

### Conclusions

11. The above data suggests that the recent growth of the private sector has produced a more even distribution of facilities in England. A significant number of district health authorities now have the opportunity to enter into co-operative arrangements with the private sector. These opportunities are more extensive if the private facilities in neighbouring districts are also taken into account. This wider availability of private facilities presents further opportunities for tendering by health authorities for contracted provision of treatment.

## Hospital Ownership, Size and Service Provision

12. The expansion in private hospital provision during the period 1979 to 1985 as well as significantly affecting the regional provision of facilities was also characterised by a change in the size and ownership of hospitals and the range of services offered. The total market provision of private acute beds can be divided between two main sectors:

### (1) Charitable Sector:

| | |
|---|---|
| Religious: | Hospitals owned or administered by religious orders. |
| Charitable: | Single hospitals registered as charities. |
| Charitable Groups: | Charities operating a number of hospitals. |

(2) **For Profit Sector:**

American Groups: Hospitals owned or operated either via subsidiaries or directly by American, investor owned companies.

British Groups: Hospitals owned or operated via subsidiaries or directly by British companies

Independents: Single hospitals owned and operated by registered companies.

13. Table 5 shows the contribution of these two sectors to the growth in private acute hospital provision between 1979 and 1985. The most noticeable trend during this time has been the increasing importance of the 'for profit' institutions which have expanded by 70 per cent over the six-year period in the number of private hospitals provided. The charitable sector has only expanded by some 4·7 per cent in the same period.

14. Table 6 shows the number of beds provided by the different sectors and sub-groups within each sector. The for profit sector again shows the fastest rate of growth during the six-year period, having grown by 163 per

TABLE 5. *Private Sector Acute Hospital Growth by Ownership Sector*

| Ownership Category | 1979 | 1985 | % Growth by Sector |
|---|---|---|---|
| **Charitable** | | | |
| Religious | 33 | 29 | |
| Charitable | 21 | 26 | |
| Charitable Groups | 30 | 33 | |
| Sub-Total | 84 | 88 | 4·7 |
| **For profit** | | | |
| American Groups | 3 | 24 | |
| British Groups | 4 | 30 | |
| Independent | 52 | 46 | |
| Sub-total | 59 | 100 | 70.0 |
| Total | 143 | 188 | |

*Sources:* AIH and Grant Thornton.
*Note:* Data is for the UK.

TABLE 6. *Private Sector Provision of Beds 1979–85*

| Ownership Category | 1979 | 1985 | % Growth by Sector |
|---|---|---|---|
| **Charitable** | | | |
| Religious | 1879 | 1761 | |
| Charitable | 1624 | 1972 | |
| Charitable Groups | 1029 | 1385 | |
| Sub-total | 4532 | 5118 | 13 |
| **For profit** | | | |
| American Groups | 366 | 1926 | |
| British Groups | 156 | 1319 | |
| Independent | 1279 | 1490 | |
| Sub-total | 1801 | 4735 | 163 |
| Total | 6333 | 9853 | |
| Average beds per hospital | 44·3 | 52·4 | |

*Sources:* AIH and Grant Thornton.

cent since 1979. Table 6 also shows that the additional hospitals provided by the for profit and the expansion of existing facilities by the charitable sector has led to an increase of approximately eight in the average number of beds per hospital.

15. Figure 1 shows an analysis of published data concerning the range of facilities provided by 42 of the 64 new hospitals opened by the for profit sector during 1979 to 1985. Although this analysis does not include all the new hospitals and may be biased towards the larger groups, it indicates the scope of services and facilities available in recently developed hospitals.

**Conclusion**

16. These findings suggest that the recent growth history of the private sector has resulted largely from the expansion of facilities provided by the for profit sector with some supporting growth from the charitable group operators. The increase in available beds of 163 per cent since 1979 has been achieved by a 70 per cent growth in hospital units. By contrast the

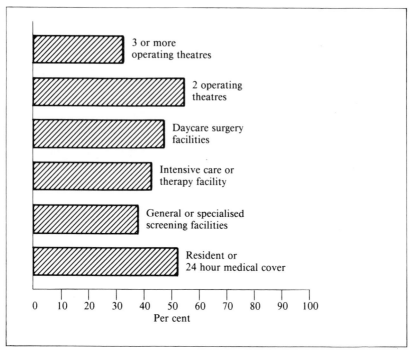

FIGURE 1. Provision of Facilities in New Hospitals Opened by the For Profit Sector
*Sample:* 42 hospitals
*Sources:* AIH, Directory of private hospitals and services (MMI), Yearbooks AIH,
IHG.

charitable sector has increased beds by 13 per cent since 1979 with a 4·7 per cent growth in hospital units. It is evident that the for profit sector has grown by opening new hospital units whilst the charitable sector has concentrated more on the expansion of existing facilities.

17. In recent years the type of hospital in the private sector has become larger and typically provides an increased range of facilities. This may well enable the scope for co-operation with the NHS to be expanded both in the provision of general surgical procedures and in specific forms of health care provision.

# CHAPTER 6

# Specific Service Provision by the Private Sector

## Introduction

1. The conclusions reached in the previous chapter suggest that the private sector is now of sufficient size to make a contribution to co-operative arrangements in the field of elective surgery. The study team decided that while these factors were important, it would also be useful to examine the potential for co-operation in certain key support services in the private sector such as pathology, pharmacy and X-ray.

2. The aim of examining these treatment support activities was to identify specific service areas where co-operation between the NHS and private sector is already in existence in order to provide an indication of the scope for future development. To do this, the study team, with the co-operation of the Independent Hospital Group, undertook a survey of a small sample of private hospitals. The details of the survey and its results are described in this chapter.

## Summary of Conclusions

3. The main conclusions concerning the service areas studied are summarised below, with further details being given in the paragraphs indicated.

(1) **Pathology** (Paragraphs 7–10)

The private hospitals sampled are already purchasing significant volumes of pathology service from the NHS. In the sample reviewed, the NHS was the largest single supplier, and most hospitals used the NHS service rather than set up their own in-house service. There thus appears to be a substantial element of buying and selling of this service, with the NHS as the major supplier.

(2) **Pharmacy** (Paragraphs 11–13)

There is a large and well developed market for the provision of pharmacy services outside the NHS and private hospital sector (i.e. wholesalers and dispensing pharmacists). This external market provides a significant volume of pharmacy service to the private sector. The extent of present NHS and private sector co-operation in this service is therefore only occasional and limited in scope.

(3) **X-ray diagnostic and treatment services** (Paragraphs 14–16)

The in-house provision of diagnostic X-ray is the main source of this service in the private sector but there is also some buying of services from the NHS. Private sector selling of diagnostic X-ray services was less in evidence, although a number of arrangements for the provision of specific procedures were quoted. There is thus evidence of a two way flow of purchase and sale of diagnostic X-ray between the two sectors. For X-ray treatment services the evidence provided by the survey was inconclusive.

# Data Collection

4. To collect suitable data on the private sector's purchase and sale of services, the study team undertook a survey of a sample of private hospitals. A questionnaire was developed in collaboration with the Independent Hospital Group (IHG) and sent to their membership. Two hundred and twenty questionnaires were sent out and seventy completed examples were returned, giving a response rate of 32 per cent. All the completed questionnaires received were from acute hospitals consistent with the definition given in Chapter 5.

5. Whilst the sample size is small in relation to the total number of private acute hospitals, it nevertheless provides an indication of the way in which private acute hospitals source these services. The sample covered different sizes of hospital and covered all ownership categories.

6. The questionnaire dealt with the following treatment support services:

(1) **Pathology services:** Respondents were asked whether they had available an in house pathology service or whether they used other

sources for the provision of the service or as a supplement. Information about the degree to which pathology was provided to the NHS was also requested.

(2) **Pharmacy services:** Information on whether the hospital employed a registered pharmacist was requested as a means of defining the availability of an in-house service. Alternative sources of pharmacy services were also assessed as well as the extent of supply of the service to the NHS.

(3) **X-ray facilities:** The availability of in-house diagnostic and treatment facilities was tested as well as the use of and provision to the NHS of both forms of service.

## Pathology Service

7. Figure 2 shows that 42 per cent of respondents to the questionnaire already had an in-house pathology service. The remaining 58 per cent sourced the service in a variety of forms involving three main types of supplier.

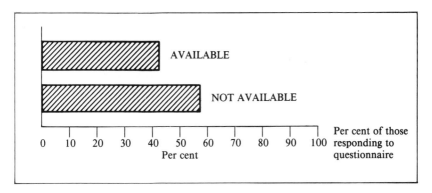

FIGURE 2. Pathology Service Available In-House.
*Sources:* Grant Thornton and IHG.

8. Figure 3 shows that 60 per cent of those respondents without an in-house pathology service obtained the service from the NHS. Commercial

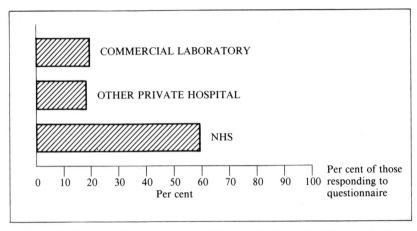

FIGURE 3. Source of Pathology Service Where no In-House Facilities Available. *Sources:* Grant Thornton and IHG.

laboratories and other private hospitals were also quoted as suppliers although the NHS was used more regularly by the majority of respondents.

9. Alternative sources of pathology services were also used by those hospitals which had an in-house provision. Figure 4 shows the frequency of the regular and occasional use of the different sources. In this case regular arrangements were less frequent than occasional arrangements as only one-third of respondents in this group had a 'regular' arrangement with any one of the three sources mentioned.

**Conclusion**

10. The above findings suggest that:

(1) Whilst a considerable percentage of private hospitals have an in house pathology service the NHS appears to be an important provider of the service to the private sector.

(2) The variety of external sources of pathology services available and

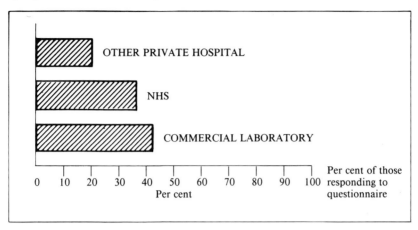

FIGURE 4. Source of Additional Service Where In-House Pathology Available. *Sources:* Grant Thornton and IHG.

used, both regularly and occasionally, by the private sector indicates that a large number of buying and selling arrangements already exist for this service.

(3) Regular arrangements or agreements with any one provider were less in evidence where in-house facilities already existed. For the occasional need for additional services the commercial laboratories supplied the main proportion of the market needs.

## Pharmacy Services

11. To establish the extent of provision of pharmacy services by the private sector respondents were asked in the questionnaire whether they employed a registered pharmacist and if not from which source they obtained their pharmacy service. Figure 5 shows that 36 per cent of respondents employed a full- or part-time registered pharmacist in-house.

12. Figure 6 shows the source of pharmacy services for those respondents who did not employ a registered pharmacist. In this case 68 per cent of respondents obtained the service through an arrangement with a local dispensing pharmacy. The 'other source' category (18 per cent) included

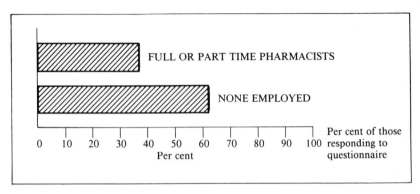

FIGURE 5. Employment of Registered Pharmacists.
*Sources:* Grant Thornton and IHG.

direct supply from wholesaler with non-pharmacist staff being responsible for ordering and control. In these cases the source of drug and prescribing advice was not evident.

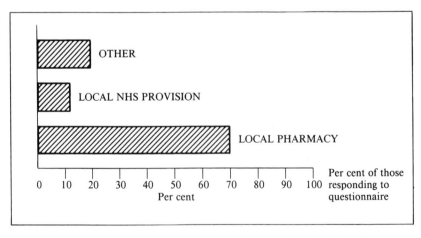

FIGURE 6. Source of Pharmacy Where Pharmacist Not Employed.
*Sources:* Grant Thornton and IHG.

**Conclusions**

13. The above findings suggest that:

(1) A minority of private hospitals in the sample provided a pharmacy service employing registered staff.

(2) The well developed and large retail market for pharmacy services is the major source for those hospitals without an in-house facility.

(3) The NHS provides a small proportion of pharmacy service needs to the private sector sampled by the questionnaire.

(4) Further discussions held with both sectors by the study team revealed that a number of formal and informal arrangements exist for the supply of pharmaceutical services in the event of emergencies, 'stock outs' and special needs. The obvious differences in scale of the NHS and the private sectors results in this exchange being predominently from the NHS to the private sector.

## X-ray Diagnosis and Treatment Services

14. Figure 7 shows that 85 per cent of respondents to the questionnaire had available in-house facilities for diagnostic procedures using X-rays. The provision of X-ray treatment facilities was shown by 32 per cent of respondents.

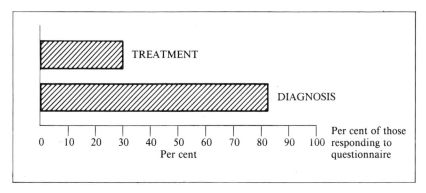

FIGURE 7. Availability of X-ray Diagnosis and Treatment Facilities
*Sources:* Grant Thornton and IHG.

15. Figure 8 shows that 67 per cent of those respondents with diagnostic X-ray facilities also made use of NHS facilities on a regular or occasional basis. However, only 10 per cent of those with in house facilities provided a service to the NHS regularly or occasionally.

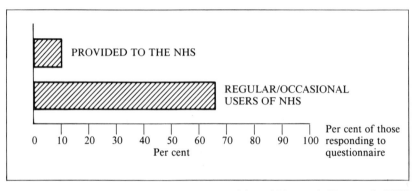

FIGURE 8. Use of NHS Diagnostic X-ray and Provision of Diagnostic X-ray to the NHS. *Sources:* Grant Thornton and IHG.

**Conclusions**

16. The above findings suggest that:

(1) The wide availability of diagnostic X-ray facilities shown in Figure 7 demonstrates the importance of this service as an integral part of acute medical care in the private sector.

(2) Considerable use of NHS facilities is also made by those private hospitals with an in house diagnostic capability. This use was defined as regular or occasional. The questionnaire did not attempt to identify whether this usage was by long-term contract or agreement or on a case-by-case basis. The level of utilisation of NHS X-ray facilities by private hospitals with their own resources may reflect a more limited scope of procedures available with the equipment in private hospitals.

(3) The relatively small amount of diagnostic X-ray provided by the private sector to the NHS is noticeable when the wide availability of resources in the private sector sample is taken into account.

(4) The small number of X-ray treatment facilities available in the private sector sample reflects the specialised nature of such services. There was little other evidence about this sevice collected from the questionnaire and no conclusions can be drawn.

(5) Unlike the pathology and pharmacy services previously examined the lack of any external third party providers of both diagnostic and treatment X-ray services suggests that collaborative and contractual arrangements in service development will be between the NHS and the private acute hospital sector.

# CHAPTER 7

# Private Sector Developments

## Introduction

1. In the previous two chapters of Part II of the report the overall size and range of services offered by the private sector have been considered. The general conclusion was reached that although the total size of the private sector is small in relation to total NHS resources, it was nevertheless of sufficient size to enable a policy of co-operation to be initiated.

2. It is not the purpose of this report to deal with the general projected growth of the private sector. However, two factors concerning its growth which have relevance in the context of developing co-operation between the two sectors are discussed in this chapter, namely:

(1) The encouragement of selected growth areas in the private sector.

(2) The regulation of the private sector.

## The Encouragement of Selected Growth Areas

3. At present, the existence of co-operative arrangements between the two sectors is at too low a level to have any material effect on the private sector market. If a general policy of co-operation was adopted by the NHS and was actively pursued, the effect on the private sector market appears likely to be:

(1) Some expansion in the total market in which the private sector could operate.

(2) An increase in competition arising from increased NHS activities in the market, particularly in relation to pay beds.

4. Within this general pattern, it is useful to consider whether encouragement should be given to certain segments of the market to grow in ways

which would be particularly relevant to the development of co-operative arrangements. The use of longer term planning arrangements between authorities and private groups may well be a useful means for achieving this. Some general examples of possible aspects where it might be useful to encourage the market to develop are listed below:

(1) The private sector is not evenly distributed throughout the U.K. Government might wish to consider the encouragement and assistance they might be able to give the private sector to develop in regions where there are few private hospitals in order to enable a policy of co-operation to be adopted more widely.

(2) Certain types of co-operative arrangement may well be found to be more useful than others. For example, in particular types of treatment where high cost capital assets can be shared. It would be useful to assess what action could be taken by health authorities and by central government to encourage the private sector to put resources into these kinds of activity so that they are available for co-operative ventures.

(3) The development of new ideas, and new ways of providing health care is important and is to be encouraged. New concepts may arise through thinking about co-operation arrangements, and may arise through the private sector developing market opportunities. The incidence of taxation in relation to private health insurance and assessment of benefits on individuals can be a highly significant factor in the development of new ideas and new approaches. It may be advisable to consider where it would be useful to encourage the development of new aspects of the market by means of taxation policy. For example, care of the elderly, and the development of health management organisations might be suitable topics for investigation in this context.

(4) Data given in the previous chapters shows that for certain conditions the private sector is already playing a significant part in the provision of elective surgery. It might be useful to encourage the further development of these specialisations by authorities entering into longer term contracts with the private sector for treatment in these specialist areas.

(5) The use of competitive tendering in relation to waiting lists has already been mentioned in this report. The adoption of a general

policy of competitive tendering relating to certain specialisations or to waiting lists generally could be used as a means for encouraging growth in those particular specialisations and for encouraging competition in the health sector generally.

(6) The form of arrangement known as franchising is an interesting form of arrangement which does not appear to have been tried in health care. It could have a useful role to play in those services where a health authority could award private operators a franchise to provide the service according to defined criteria. For example, health screening might be the kind of service where franchising might be applied, possibly on the basis that the franchisee could make a charge to individuals. Franchising should be considered as an area where it might be useful to stimulate private sector growth.

# Regulation of the Private Sector

5. There is a need for any industry or service to maintain the confidence of the consumer. Where health is concerned, clearly the consumer must have total confidence in the provider. At the present time, the private health sector would generally be judged to enjoy an extremely high level of confidence and nothing in the present study has indicated otherwise. Even so, if the market is to open up in the way indicated, with possibly new operators joining it, it may well be advisable for the private sector to take steps to ensure that this confidence level is maintained and that it has the mechanism available to do so. If, for example, general confidence in the private sector was for any reason to fall, it would become difficult for the NHS to enter into co-operation arrangements, and that important new segment of the market for the private sector would not develop.

### The present arrangements for regulation

6. Many sectors of the economy require some form of regulation regarding quality, operating standards and other matters. Sectors offering services to individual consumers may well tend to have close regulation which protects the individual consumer, but which equally importantly, protects all the operators in the service by not allowing the service to

develop a poor reputation through the poor standards of a few operators. Regulation may be provided by a government body, or it may be self-regulation provided by a representative body of the operators themselves.

7. At present, in the private health sector, regulation of hospitals is provided by the local health authorities, carrying out the responsibility placed on them by legislation. There is no form of self-regulation provided by the private hospital sector itself.

8. The regulation provided by health authorities takes the form of requiring the registration of premises, and the regular inspection of those premises. Recently, comprehensive guidelines have been issued to health authorities relating to the registration and inspection of private sector premises, and providing model guidelines relating to the standards to be applied (Registration and Inspection of Nursing Homes, National Association of Health Authorities in England and Wales). These guidelines should assist the application of standard principles of regulation throughout the country, although of course each health authority has to interpret them in relation to local conditions.

9. In broad terms the regulations imposed by legislation and applied by local health authorities deal principally with what might be called the physical and technical aspects of hospitals and nursing homes. For example, in the case of acute private hospitals the regulations deal with the facilities required in an operating suite, and its size, structure, ventilation and lighting. There are, however, other matters, which are not physical or technical but which can be equally important to control if the quality of private sector service and reputation are to be maintained. These quality of service standards may well be best operated by the sector itself on a self-regulatory basis. It is suggested that the private health sector might wish to consider this aspect of self-regulation as a means of ensuring its quality in a growing market.

**Aspects of self-regulation in the private health sector**

10. Self-regulation in business and professional sectors is normally applied by setting up an association of members which then develops a series of published operating standards. Only organisations conforming

to these standards can be accredited as members of the association, and the association needs to develop some means for monitoring that members are adhering to the agreed code of conduct. Although it is understood that some self-regulation of this kind is carried out, it could be usefully developed further by the private hospital sector.

11. To do this, it would be necessary to clarify the roles of the various associations which currently represent the sector, possibly, with a view to merger or it might be necessary to create a new association for the purpose.

12. The regulations to be applied in the private hospital sector would be developed by the association and their content would depend on its members' views. Listed below is a summary of those aspects which might be considered:

(1) **Physical/technical aspects.** Although minimum physical and technical aspects are dealt with by the government regulations, it may be that the private sector wishes to apply higher or more comprehensive standards, or to develop a series of standards for various categories of private sector hospitals.

(2) **Financial standing.** In many sectors, the financial standing of members is an important part of self-regulation. Although perhaps of less relevance in the health sector, self-regulation requirements could usefully be applied relating to audit, accounts and ability to finance and maintain the level of services provided.

(3) **Range and quality of services.** The study showed that there is a very wide range in the facilities and services provided in-house by private hospitals. It may well be that a self-regulatory system could usefully provide standards for the type, range and source of services required for different categories of hospital.

(4) **Company ownership.** A useful matter for self-regulation may well be the question of company structure, and ownership. Self-regulation might usefully be developed concerning the ownership of hospitals, such as the circumstances in which hospitals and health insurance organisations may be under common ownership and the circumstances in which consultants may refer patients to a hospital in which

the consultant has some degree of ownership. With the likely development of new approaches to private health care in the future, the ownership of the businesses and their interrelationships may well be an important aspect of self-regulation.

(5) **Legal arrangements.** The contractual relationships between patient and hospital may be another useful area for self-regulation. Standards might be defined for the form of contract between hospital and patient, and for the procedures to be followed where complaints arise. Indemnity insurance levels could also be defined.

# PART III

# Programme and Conclusion

# CHAPTER 8

# A Suggested Programme

## Introduction

1. The proposals for the development of co-operation between the two sectors in the way described in this report will require careful consideration and implementation over a period of time. Summarised in this chapter is a suggested logical order in which certain general steps might be taken towards implementation, and indicating in particular those areas where it may be possible to take steps in the immediate future.

## Immediate Developments

2. The developments where consideration should be given to taking action in the short-term, as a means of encouraging the development of co-operative arrangements are summarised below:

(1) **Legislation.** There will be a number of areas where it will be necessary for changes in legislation or NHS regulations to be made to enable health authorities to enter into commercial arrangements with the private sector, to set up operating companies or trusts and to make investments in joint venture organisations. If a policy of further co-operation with the private sector is to be adopted, it is suggested that a study into the legislation changes required should be initiated now.

(2) **Appointment of commercial managers.** The appointment of commercial managers to be responsible to health authority general managers for the development of NHS commercial activities and for co-operation with the private sector was suggested in a previous chapter. There would appear to be no reason why authorities should not now consider making such appointments.

(3) **Segregation of revenue earning activities.** The creation of subsidiary companies or trusts to deal with long-term revenue earning activities

of health authorities has been discussed in a previous chapter. The setting up of such organisations could be carried out independently of the other proposed changes in financial arrangements and, subject to legislation, it would be useful for that to be done as soon as possible.

(4) **Inter authority charging systems.** The nature of an internal market for buying and selling services within the NHS was discussed in a previous chapter. The operation of such a market will require the development of transfer payment systems for services and patients. There is no reason why such systems for services could not be introduced now, and authorities might find it useful to consider doing so. For patients, although the full development of transfer payment systems may be a matter for longer term development, there would appear to be no reason why interim transfer payment arrangements for particular types of patient might not be introduced now, based on estimated costs.

(5) **Competitive tendering for patient care.** It might be useful for authorities to consider using competitive tendering as a means of dealing with specific patient waiting lists, obtaining quotations from both the private sector and from other NHS hospitals as well from an in-house bid. An initiative of this kind might provide a useful way to reduce waiting lists and to encourage wider co-operation between the two sectors, and to initiate the internal market concept.

(6) **Contract management of NHS hospitals.** The use of private sector management to manage an NHS pay bed activity or an NHS hospital along the lines suggested in the Trust's handbook *Developing co-operation between public and private hospitals* would be a major step in introducing the concept of buying and selling services between the two sectors. It could be introduced in the short-term, possibly in the context of a new hospital.

(7) **Encouragement of growth areas.** Consideration should be given to the action needed by the public health sector to encouraging the areas of private sector growth described in Chapter 7 as a means of expanding the scope for co-operation.

# Longer Term Developments

3. A number of the suggested developments in the NHS financial arrangements could not be introduced in the immediate future as it will take time to design and implement the necessary bases and systems of accounting. It would however, be advisable to make a start on the development work as soon as possible, in particular:

(1) **Self accounting arrangements.** The setting up of self accounting arrangements in the form of income and expenditure statements and balance sheets to replace the present final financial statements of authorities will require a considerable amount of development work, including some revision of the financial responsibilities placed on authorities. It would be advisable to start work now to define the nature of these responsibilities and to define the principles on which the revised form of accounts is to be based.

(2) **Asset accounting.** The need for full asset accounting in the NHS has been dealt with in a previous chapter. It will be necessary for asset accounting to be in operation, at least in provisional form before full self accounting by authorities could be introduced. The development and implementation of full asset accounting procedures would be the task requiring the longest lead time in the proposed developments and it would be advisable for it to be initiated now.

4. Regarding the private sector, the main development required for the longer term is the proposed use of self-regulation as a means of maintaining the standards of the sector. It would be useful now to initiate discussion relating to the structure of a self-regulatory body and its method of working.

# CHAPTER 9

# Conclusion

---

1. This report has dealt with the more fundamental issues relating to the development of co-operation between the two sectors. It has set out in broad terms what would need to be done in both sectors if the buying and selling of services between them is to be developed into a more dynamic form of market than the present *ad-hoc* use of co-operation arrangements.

2. This report has, however, dealt only with the broader issues. More detailed, practical, matters have been dealt with in the Trust's handbook *Developing co-operation between public and private hospitals.* That book deals with the nature of contracting, the way in which risk is shared, and the use of contracts for patient treatment and hospital management. It includes a number of case studies, and attempts to set out a best practice for management in seeking and setting up contracts between the two sectors.

3. Looking to the future, the report has suggested the main steps which would be needed to implement a policy of co-operation. It has placed particular emphasis on the important changes which would be needed in the financial and management arrangements at health authorities to enable them to operate in a more flexible way in relation to the private sector. It has stressed that these important changes are essential if health authorities are to develop improved management control over their assets and resources.

4. The report has also emphasised the need for the private sector to develop its regulatory procedures, not because of any adverse comments received about the sector's present activities, but because without a stronger basis of self-regulation the sector may well find difficulty in maintaining standards in its future growth.